Live Life Well! Survival Guide

By Lori R. Vargas, MBA, CPA

Special Thanks to Ann M. Babiarz for earlier collaborations that had a great influence on this survival guide.

Live Life Well! Survival Guide

Table of Contents

Introduction to Live Life Well - Survival Guide

What does Live Life Well really mean? Do you really need a survival guide? ***Live Life Well! Survival Guide*** is a resource to assist you on your path to improved health and fitness. The mantra of Live Life Well is a commitment to yourself and one that needs to be embraced on a daily basis. This survival guide will encourage, cultivate and promote optimal fitness, healthy eating and balanced living. The goal of the guide is to inspire all people to live happy and healthy lives. The guide will provide you with a framework to establish your personal nutrition and exercise plans. The plans that you establish will be bio-individual and need to align with your goals, values, beliefs, culture and schedule.

Fitness means good health, especially good physical condition resulting from exercise and proper nutrition. Optimal fitness is the best health to condition and fuel the body! On a daily basis, we are making daily choices that influence our way of life. Lifestyle choices are choices a person makes about how to live and behave, according to one's attitudes, tastes and values. Fitness is a lifestyle choice that each individual must define; it is bio-individual.

The desire to change your lifestyle will influence what steps you need to take to achieve your goals. The desired changes could be to increase your energy level or reduce your stress level. You may want to change your body composition or gain/lose weight. You may want to create a better balance of life.

The objective is to empower yourself and optimize your energy to live a balanced, healthier and fuller life every day.

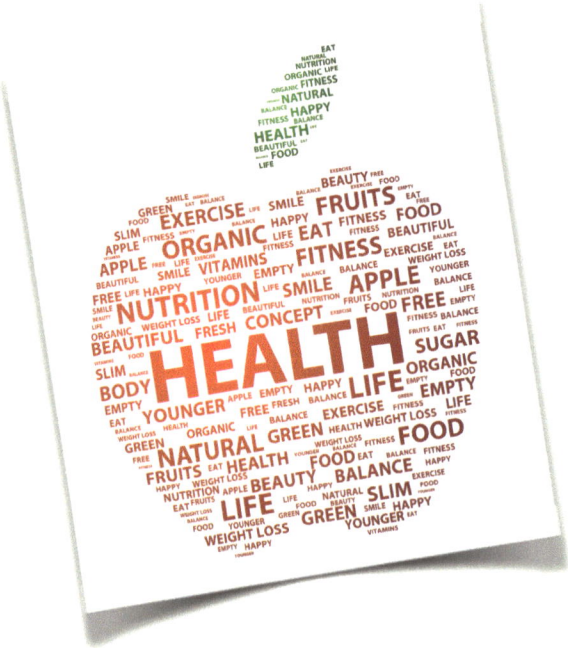

4

Health & Fitness Assessment

What is **your** optimal fitness? What is **your** optimal nutrition? What is **your** ideal body shape? The media has a strong influence on what is "ideal" in our culture. Equally, relationships have an impact on how we feel about ourselves. It is time for you to define what your health goals are for yourself and your family. The following questions and chart will allow you to gain insight to what is important to you and will be used to track your success. Complete everything objectively and candidly. This survival guide is for your personal growth and journaling. Once you establish what you want to achieve, the next step will be to establish a plan to make it happen!

Health and Fitness Survey

- What do you want to change about your current lifestyle?
    - Eat more heart-healthy, nutrient-rich foods
    - Establish a consistent weekly exercise program
    - Lose, gain or tone body
    - Improve sleeping habits
    - Lower stress level
    - _____
- What are your nutrition goals?
    - Improve eating habits
    - Eat more vegetables and fruits
    - Eat more lean proteins
    - Improve your culinary skills and eat at home more
    - Design a health-encouraging kitchen
    - Eliminate or reduce sugar and salt
    - Eliminate or reduce processed foods
    - _____
- What are your primary motivators in changing your body composition?
    - Lower heart and diabetes risk
    - Lower stress levels
    - Lose or gain a stated amount of pounds; fat not muscle
    - Fit into your skinny jeans
    - _____
- What has been successful for you in reaching weight changing goals in the past?
    - Volumize by eating low calorie-density food
    - Increase water intake
    - Calorie counting
    - Eliminating food categories
    - Adding or increasing exercise frequency and intensity
    - _____

Health and Fitness Survey

- What are your exercise goals?
    - To lower risk of lifestyle diseases
    - To improve cardio or build strength and/ or tone muscles
    - Weight control
    - To age gracefully
    - To reduce stress levels
    - _____

- How often do you exercise current?
    - Never
    - 1-3 times a week
    - 4-5 times a week

- What type of exercise do you participate in?
    - _____
    - _____

- How is your nutrition?
    - I am a junkfood junkie
    - I have no time so prepared foods or eating out is my approach
    - Whatever I crave it, I eat it
    - I cook most of my meals
    - I fuel my body with healthy clean food
    - _____

- Do you crave any of the following foods
    - Chocolate
    - Salt
    - Sugar
    - Caffeine
    - _____

- How much sleep do you get on a nightly basis?
    - 4 hours or less
    - 5 to 6 hours a night
    - 7 to 8 hours a night
    - 9 or more hours a night

- What is your stress level?
    - Minimal stress
    - Moderate stress
    - Extreme stress

- What is stopping you from reaching your goals?
    - Time, I have no time to change
    - Desire, I don't want to change current lifestyle
    - Stress
    - Money, I perceive the changes will cost more money that I do not have
    - Not able to be consistent with change in my life
    - _____

6

MEASUREMENT TRACKER

	Day 1	Day 30	Day 60	Day 90	Day 120	Target
Weight						
Height						
Body Mass Index						
Bust						
Chest						
Waist						
Hips						
Thighs						
Calves						
Upper Arm						
Forearm						

Body Mass Index Guidelines

Underweight	Less than 18.5%
Healthy	18.5% - 24%
Overweight	25% - 29%
Obese	30% or more

Document your current body metrics in the tracking grid above in Day 1 and complete the Target column. It is important to have measurable goals that are monitored on a frequent basis. The targets need to be realistic and reasonable. This form of tracking is meant to be motivating. If you find that the Measurement Tracker is not aiding you in accomplishing your goals then skip this process.

Achieving the After

"Before and After" pictures are great sources of motivation – we all want to be the "after model" but many times feel like we are a shoe-in for the "before model." Keep reminding yourself when you look at magazines – it is their job to be in top shape. It is important to start taking care of your body vessel in a healthy manner. Take pictures of yourself to document where you are, full body front and side are great benchmark pictures.

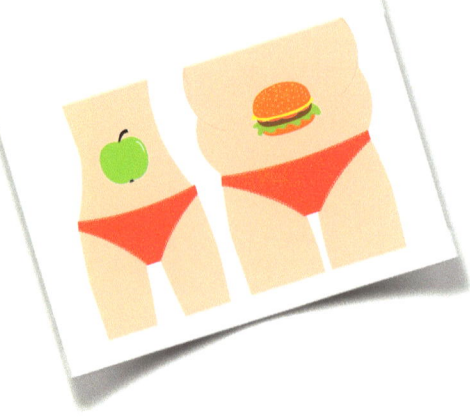

Are you tired of being what you consider, too fat or too skinny? Are you concerned about the risk to your heart or for diabetes? It's time to imagine waking up, gazing at yourself in the mirror, and actually being ecstatic and amazed about what you see! This is possible. With the right choices, you have the ability to create the body you want and be in the health you desire. It is time to make movement toward your goals.

Another obstacle that is rarely discussed is how our self talk hinders our progress in change. Self talk is the internal voice inside your head that determines how you perceive every situation. Many times this self talk is influenced by beliefs that may not be accurate information. Illustrated are a few common beliefs that are not accurate but may be sabotaging your efforts.

Belief: Fad diets work for permanent weight loss. Key word is PERMANENT.

Truth: Fad diets are not the best way to lose weight and keep it off. If they did work, there wouldn't be so many of them. Fad diets will often promise quick weight loss or tell you to cut certain foods from your diets. Diets that strictly limit calories or food choices are hard to follow and most people tire of them very quickly. What happens? They regain what they lost and often times more!

To top it off, fad diets may not include all the nutrients your body needs. Not to mention that weight loss at a rapid rate may increase your risk for developing gallstones or more serious health conditions. For example, cutting your calories to below 800 calories per day could also result in heart rhythm abnormalities, which can be fatal.

Focus Point: Research suggests that losing ½ to 2 pounds a week by making healthy food choices, eating moderate portions, and building physical activities into your daily life is the best way to lose weight and keep it off. By adopting healthy habits, you may also lower your risk for developing type 2 diabetes, heart disease, and high blood pressure.

Belief: High protein/low-carbohydrate diets are a healthy way to lose weight.

Truth: The long-term health effects of a high-protein/low carbohydrate diet are unknown. Obtaining most of your nutrition from high-protein foods like meat, eggs and cheese is not a balanced eating plan.

Eating fewer than 130 grams of carbohydrate a day can lead to a buildup of ketones in your blood. Ketones are partially broken down fats and a buildup of ketones in your blood can cause your body to produce high levels of uric acid, which is a risk factor for gout and kidney stones.

Focus Point: High-protein/low-carbohydrate diets are often low in calories because food choices are strictly limited, so they may cause short-term weight loss. A reduced-calorie eating plan that includes recommended amounts of carbohydrate, protein, and fat will also allow you to lose weight. By following a balanced eating plan, you will not have to stop eating whole categories of foods. You may also find it easier to stick with an eating plan where moderation is the norm.

Belief: Certain foods, like grapefruit, celery, or cabbage soup, can burn fat and make you lose weight.

Truth: No foods can burn fat. Some foods with caffeine may speed up your metabolism, for a short time, but they do not cause weight loss.

Focus Point: The best way to lose weight is to cut back on the number of calories you eat, especially "empty" calories and be physically active.

Belief: Natural or herbal weight-loss products are safe and effective.

Truth: A weight-loss product that claims to be "natural" or "herbal" is not necessarily safe. These products are not usually scientifically tested to prove that they are safe or that they work. For example, herbal products containing ephedra, now banned by the U.S. FDA, have caused serious health problems and even death. Newer products that claim ephedra free are not necessarily danger-free.

Focus Point: Talk with your health care provider before using any weight-loss product. Some natural or herbal weight-loss products can be harmful.

Belief: Skipping meals is a good way to lose weight.

Truth: Studies show that people who skip breakfast and eat fewer times during the day tend to be heavier than people who eat a healthy breakfast and eat four or five times daily. This may be because people who skip meals tend to feel hungrier later on, and eat more than they normally would. It may also be that eating many small meals throughout the day helps people control their appetites.

Focus Point: Eat smaller meals throughout the day that include a variety of healthy, low-fat, low-calorie foods. This is the recommended approach!

Belief: Eating after 8 p.m. causes weight gain.

Truth: It does not matter what time of day you eat. It is what and how much you eat and how much physical activity you do that determines whether you gain, lose, or maintain your weight. No matter when you eat, your body will store extra calories as fat.

Focus Point: If you want to have a snack before bedtime, think first about how many calories you have eaten that day. Try to avoid snacking in front of the TV at night, it may be easier to overeat when you are distracted by the television.

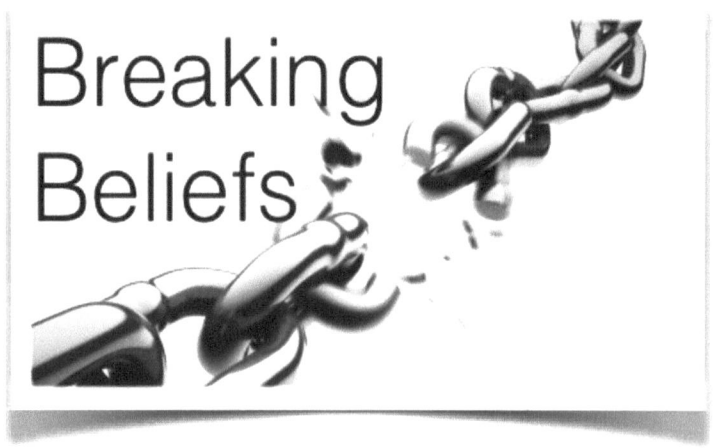

FOR CHANGE - YOU MUST CHANGE! LIFESTYLE CHANGES!

Nutrition, fitness and sleep all are factors that influence your health and the condition of your well-being. And extremely important is the knowledge that each of these variables IS influenced and controlled by YOU. So, if you truly want to change it is up to only YOU to make the change happen. The goal is to be physically fit, have a balanced nutritional intake and good sleep habits that nurture your body!

The answers to the survey provide you insight to areas that you want or need to change. The difference between Day 1 and Target from the chart is your measurable opportunity for change. That change or movement will need a plan to achieve your goals. This guide is not intended to provide you with exact steps but will provide you with various strategies that you can select from to develop a success plan designed by you for you. From this moment on, you can expect that your mind, body and quality of life will only improve, that is, if you honor your commitments.

The First Step: Commitment

It's time to make a decision and pledge your full commitment to doing what it takes to get healthy.

Fitness experts say that you are much more likely to stick with a fitness routine if you put it in writing. One great way to do this is for you to make a contract with yourself!

So, if you're serious, put it in writing! Complete and post this contract on your refrigerator or bulletin board so you can look at it every day for inspiration. Ultimately, **you are responsible** for your own results.

With this contract, you will promise to satisfy all of the necessary commitments to help you reach your health and fitness goals. Commit to this program like you would any high-importance task at work or at home and commit to getting the most from the program.

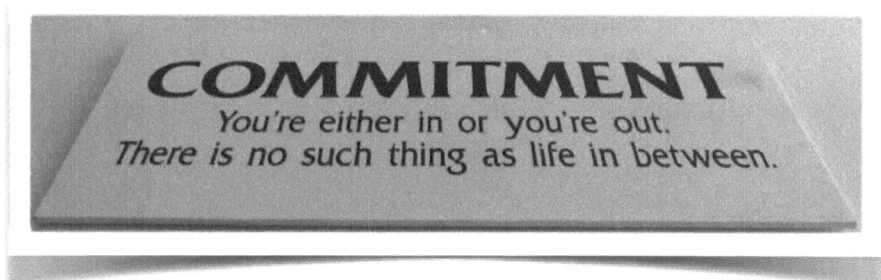

Live Life Well Commitment Contract

I, _____, promise to commit to incorporating a solid self-care program to the best of my abilities by looking at myself and my life honestly, thoroughly, and without judgment.

I promise that before I skip any of the assignments or decide to stop this program, I will reread this contract.

I promise to recognize the inevitable negative feelings and frustrations which may come up for me during the program, while recognizing and honoring them as my feelings, will not empower them by allowing them to stop or slow me down.

My Inspiration is .....

Why do I want to change?	1.
	2.
	3.
What steps do I need to take?	1.
	2.
	3.
What are my top 3 goals?	1.
	2.
	3.
How am I going to feel when I achieve my goals?	1.
	2.
	3.
What will my life look like when I obtain this goal?	1.
	2.
	3.
What are my obstacles?	1.
	2.
	3.
How will I overcome those obstacles?	1.
	2.
	3.
Who will help me or hold me accountable to my goals?	1.
	2.
	3.
When will I begin?	1.
	2.
	3.

My Inspiration is …..

When will I achieve my goal 1?	1. 2. 3.
When will I achieve my goal 2?	1. 2. 3.
When will I achieve my goal 3?	1. 2. 3.
How will I reward myself for making progress toward my goal?	1. 2. 3.

_____   _____

Signature   Date

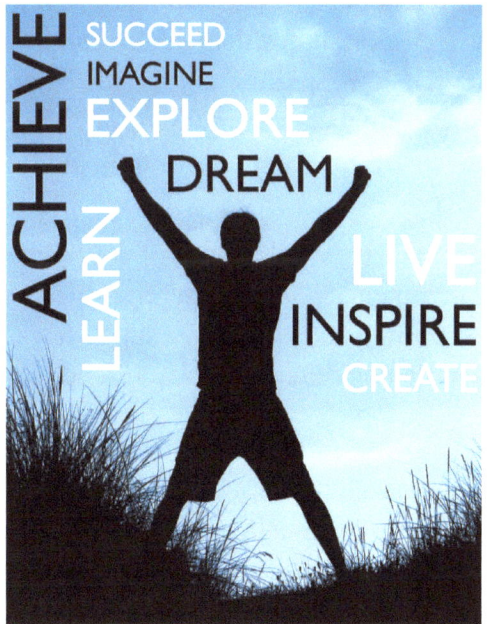

The Second Step: Optimal Nutrition

The process of eating needs to be a conscious practice starting with meal planning, shopping, preparing to consuming. The awareness to what is and is not going into your body to improve body efficiency is critical. This awareness includes substances and environmental toxins.

Optimal means the most favorable or desirable; having the most positive qualities; best. ***Nutrition*** means the process of nourishing or being nourished, the process by which a living organism assimilates food and uses it for growth and for proper health and development. ***Optimal Nutrition*** is the best nourishment to fuel the body! Proper nutrition is critical at all ages. Make the best of every meal and enjoy each meal.

If you are going to improve your health by changing your eating plan and have the goal of weight change, it is up to you! If you are discouraged, you will have a more difficult time staying with your improved meal plan. If you need a support network, get one! Make sure it is a group that is positive and supportive. A group that really stands behind healthy eating being about balance, variety and moderation rather than deprivation.

How balanced and healthy are your eating habits? What are you putting on your plate? Would you put anything in the gas tank of your automobile other than gasoline? We do this to our bodies all the time. We fill ourselves up with nutritionally worthless fuel and expect our bodies to perform at top levels. Many things play a factor in how we feel and nutrition is a significant component. Nutrition is an input to and foundation for health and development. Nutritional awareness is the understanding and satisfying your body's needs. The connection between overall health and nutrition is well documented. Better nutrition means a healthier you. It means stronger immune systems, less illness and better health. Healthy children learn better. Healthy people are stronger, are more productive and more able to create opportunities. Simply put, food = medicine.

Evaluate your plate each time you eat. Fill up half of your plate with fruits and vegetables, quarter with lean protein and quarter with whole grains. This quick approach is an easy starting point on your pursuit to healthy eating. Avoid food which promote inflammation. Incorporate food in your meal plan that are anti-inflammatory.

Meal planning is important on a weekly basis. Select a weekly preparation day to prepare foods for the week. Time saving tip is to cook meals for two dinners and enough leftovers to make your next day lunch. Pack your lunch the night before so it is ready for you in the morning. This will ensure that you have a balanced lunch and that you are in control of your nutrition.

As individuals, it makes sense for us to strive for great health and longevity as well as to serve as an example to our children by following proper nutritional habits. For example, each time you eat it is your choice on what you do or what you don't put in your body.

14

Each time you shop for food, it is you deciding what food choices are going to be available in your household. You have the responsibility to yourself and your family to improve your food selections to assure that everyone has sound, healthy choices.

Fuel the Body

Fueling the body is a ***conscious approach*** to nourishing your body. In order to engage in a program of healthy eating and proper nutrition, you need to have the right mind-set or commitment! But equally important is that you have to be mindful and aware. No more being on auto-pilot with grocery shopping and food consumption. ***Awareness*** to what is and is not going into the body to improve body efficiency. It is time to start reading the food labels and understanding the source of your food. ***Balance*** each meal; use your plate as a guide for each meal. Fill half of your plate with fruits and vegetables, a quarter of your plate with whole grains and a quarter of your plate with lean protein. Have your intentions align with your goals and objectives.

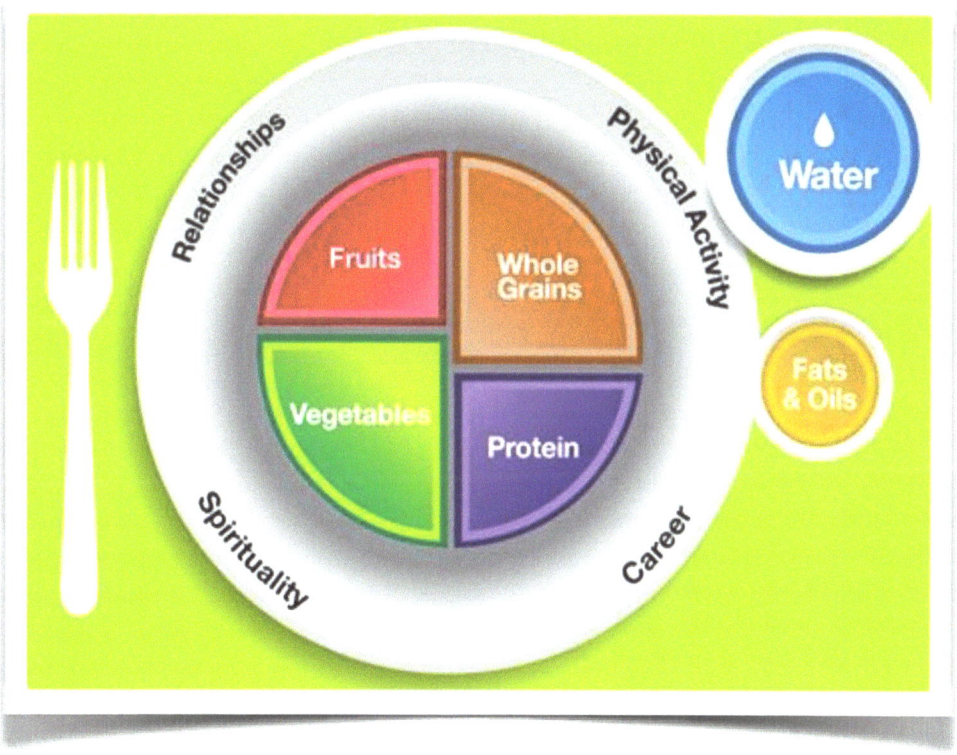

Carbohydrates are the body's most preferred source of energy and play a vital part in digestion, metabolism and oxidation of protein and fat. Unused carbohydrates are stored in the liver or converted into fat and stored in the tissues for future use.

- **Simple carbohydrate**s are quick energy sources. Sources include sugar, fruit juice, honey, soft drinks and sweets. REDUCE the intake of these sugary options.
- **Complex carbohydrates** supply energy, nutrients and fiber. Sources of starch include bread, cereal, potatoes, pasta, rice and legumes. Sources of fiber include bran, whole-grain foods, raw vegetables and fruit, legumes, nuts, seeds and popcorn. *Complex carbs are the preferred choice.*

Proteins are part of every cell, tissue and organ. Proteins are digested into amino acids that are used to replace the old protein. Sources include meats, poultry, fish, legumes, tofu, nuts and seeds and milk. *Lean protein is the preferred choice.*

Fats and oils are essential for body functions.

- **Unsaturated fats** are found in nuts, vegetable oils, avocados and fish containing omega fatty acids. *Unsaturated fats is the preferred choice.*
- **Saturated fats** are found in cheese, high fat cuts of meats, whole-fat milk, butter and ice cream, along with other processed foods.
- **Trans saturated fats** are artificially derived and impossible for the body to breakdown. Eliminate the intake of these types of fats.

Fresh Quality Ingredients

An eating regimen rich in vegetables, fruits, whole-grain and high fiber foods, fish, lean protein and low fat dairy products is the key. Knowing the source of where your food is coming from is becoming more and more important. Learning to read the food labels to understand what is in the product and how it has been raised or produced. Reduce or eliminate refined grains, processed foods, sugar and salts. Research has proven all of these consumptions are not healthy for the body.

Protein - buy grass-fed, free range, hormone-free and organic meat as often as possible. If you can't afford "best choice" meats, then select the leanest cuts and cut off the fats. This is where the antibiotics, hormones, environmental toxins and pro-inflammatory omega-6 fatty acids "live." Pastured, organic eggs are a great source of high quality protein.

Produce - the best choice is in season, local, fresh and organic. Seek produce that is pesticide free and is not genetically modified organisms (GMO). Vary your produce by color.

Whole Grains - All your grains should be **WHOLE** or cracked. Avoid refined, enriched or processed grains since they are deficient in nutrients.

Nutritional Tips to consider

Commit to eating a nutritious breakfast every morning

Stay hydrated with water to avoid confusing thirst for hunger

If you have a craving or feel hungry outside of meal time, drink 8 ounces of water and wait 10 minutes before you take a bite

Eat healthy snacks. Vegetables and low sugar fruits are great choices

Pick portion-controlled meals that have fiber and protein

The more fruits and vegetables, the better

Maximize flavor with herbs and spices

Prepare your own meals and use the healthiest ingredients whenever possible

Keep your metabolism going by eating 4-6 small meals per day

Eat healthy 90% of the time and dedicate 10% to cravings!

Top Triggers to avoid that cause mindless eating

Triggers	Tip to Overcome
Boredom	Select fruits and vegetables to snack
Feelings of Deprivation	Balance healthy eating & exercise. Balance calories in and calories out.
Body Loathing	Develop a positive self-image. Define personal values.
Glucose Intolerance	Spread your calories out by eating small amounts frequently.
Daily Habits: - Excessive Eating - Lack of Physical Activity	Break those habits! Instead of watching television, become active. Or workout while you are watching TV. Begin journaling and get your feelings on paper.
Sad or stressed	Take a walk. Breathe deeply and chill.
Comfort eating	Make time for yourself. Schedule a monthly massage at a spa!
Lack of energy or feeling tired	Substitute eating with activity.
Feeling overwhelmed	Set realistic goals so frustration does not occur!

17

Optimal Nutrition Leads to a Healthier Life

Underweight = *Unhealthy.*   Being underweight has health implications ranging from menstrual disorders to malnutrition.   Overweight = *Unhealthy.* Carrying extra weight dramatically increases chronic ailments and diseases, which are forms of malnutrition. These forms are often characterized by obesity and the long-term implications of unbalanced dietary and lifestyle practices. Poor nutritional practices result in chronic diseases such as cardiovascular disease, cancer, and diabetes.

Optimal Body Weight and Shape = *HEALTHY!*

Nutrition is the ingredient that makes the **BIGGEST** difference on weight change. Eating well will not only allow you to improve your health and energy, and it also provides the ideal environment for your transformation - maintain lean muscle while reducing unwanted fat. *If your waist is larger than your hips you have room for improvement!*

If your goal is to lose body fat and not muscle, you must eat slightly fewer calories than you burn. This may seem simple, but when calories are significantly reduced, the body becomes imbalanced. It is the body's job to restore balance, and it inevitably does so by either reducing the amount of calories it burns for energy, by using muscle instead of fat or by forcing you to eat more through hunger and cravings. This is one of the main reasons why fad diets do not produce long term results.

A change in lifestyle is key to getting and staying healthy. Some people do lose weight on diets due to water loss, eating fewer calories or a combination. Less than five percent of these dieters are able to keep the weight off permanently. Diets simply don't work long term; lifestyle changes do. Replace improper nutrition with proper nutrition and add physical activity and enjoy the benefits of wonderful, more vibrant health.

Research is showing that America is fatter as a society today. Why? We consume approximately 300 to 500 more calories per day than we did 10 years ago, yet we move less because of advances in technology such as computers, escalators and other labor-saving devices. Hmmmm, more energy in and less energy out makes for a constant overage which then translates into, you guessed it, FAT!

Proper nutrition can be mastered by understanding that everything you eat and drink can either positively or negatively affect your weight change goals. *There needs to be a conscious evolution of thought that nutrition is to fuel the body.* That is as simple as it will get. Ask yourself a few questions before you consume anything. Is this consumption properly fueling my body? Does this consumption align with my health and fitness goals?

Understand Your Food Cravings

Salty and crunchy potato chips will satisfy my cravings every time! What do you crave? Chocolate? Coffee? Alcohol? Cigarettes? Broccoli? Milk shakes? The ability to understand your hunger and letting it cue you to eat, rather than feeding your emotions is important. Become a student of your body and start understanding what your body's wants and needs mean. Cravings tend to be a nutrient deficiency in the body. Many people crave sugar, carbohydrates, or alcohol not because of eating disorders but due to unhealthy nutrition. One thing the doctors agree on, if you have dieted over a long period of time, particularly low-fat dieting, chances are your metabolism needs to heal itself first. If you become aware of your common cravings, you can do daily work to slowly change your unhealthy habits and get back to a normal lifestyle that is not controlled by physical imbalances.

When you find yourself craving a particular food,
try eating the healthy food choice in small amounts.

The good news: it is possible to get your body back into balance with the right food choices made every day and supplement only where absolutely necessary.

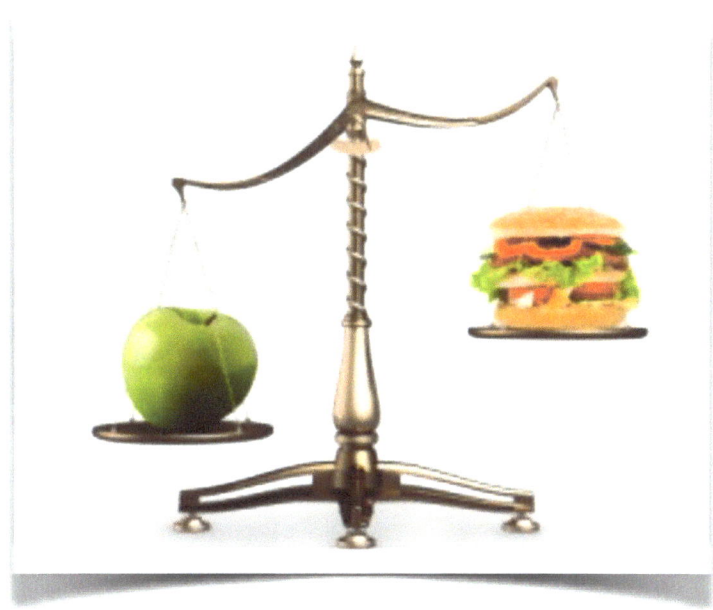

19

Top Cravings and Their Healthy Food Choices

Cravings	Reasons why..	Healthy Choices
Chocolate	Body may need magnesium or copper	Butternut squash, organic corn, apples, bananas, nuts, organic dark chocolate
Salt	Body may need healthy sodium or chloride	Celery, fish, unrefined sea salt, goat milk yogurt
Sugar	Exhausted or feeling depressed, blood sugar and serotonin levels are low	Broccoli, grapes, cheese, chicken, eggs, fresh fruits, kale, spinach, carrots, sweet potatoes
Bread	Upset, stressed, exhausted, feeling depressed, blood sugar and serotonin levels are low	Lean protein, chicken, eggs, black beans, fish
Dairy	Body may need calcium	Broccoli, kale, cheese, legumes, turnip greens
Caffeine	Body may need iron, sulfur, phosphorus and salt	Chicken, eggs, red pepper, garlic, onion, seaweed, kale, broccoli, black cherries
Ice to chew	Body may need iron	Meat, fish, poultry, seaweed, kale, spinach, red meat, black cherries

Functions Minerals and Nutrients have in the Body

Mineral or Nutrient	Function
Magnesium	Regulates muscle and nerve function, blood glucose control and blood pressure regulation
Copper	Helps make red blood cells and keeps nerve cells and your immune system healthy
Sodium	Control blood pressure and blood volume
Chloride	An electrolyte that works to ensure the body's metabolism is working correctly and essential part of digestive juices
Serotonin	Neurotransmitter responsible for maintaining mood balance
Iron	Carries oxygen from your lungs throughout the body
Sulfur	Vital amino acids used to create protein for cells and tissues; essential for maintaining youthful skin, joints and a healthy digestive system
Calcium	Most essential nutrient for bone health
Phosphorus	Mineral that provides structure and strength in the bones and teeth
Protein	Protein builds and repairs tissues and are critical in cells
Glutamine	Amino acid found in muscles
Potassium	Regulates electrolytes, nerve function, muscle control and blood pressure

Juicing is a Great Source of Nutrients

Juicing plant based food is an effective nutritionally dense approach to fuel the body. There are two techniques of juicing; extracted and blender. Extracted brings out all fresh raw juice from produce. A concentrated glass of live, pure nutrients is the highly recommended approach. The blender approach combines pulp, fiber and juice into waterless smoothies. Blending breaks down fiber for easier digestion. Some fruits do not juice well, like bananas, so blending works better.

Cleansing, detoxifying, renewing and restoring for body and mind. Sculpt your body, boost your health, renew your mind and improve your whole outlook on life. This is the preferred method of effectively fueling the body.

Supplements

Consult your physician or certified nutritionist before adding supplements to your eating plan. Supplements are alternatives of ensuring that your body gets the correct fuel to run efficiently. Proper supplementation gives your body the nutrients it needs without adding calories. Due to the way we are processing foods these days and to our busy lifestyles, it may be difficult to satisfy your body's nutritional needs with the number of calories recommended to achieve you weight change goals. By supplying the body with the natural nutrients it needs without additional calories, you can help satisfy all your nutritional needs for repair and growth without exceeding the amount of calories your body needs to maintain the mandatory deficit for weight change.

The mainstay of any fitness program is a whole food nutrient complex or multi-vitamin. You may also find that you need additional vitamins, minerals, enzymes, essential fatty acids and antioxidants that will boost your nutrient intake beyond what is available through the foods you eat. These additional nutrients allow cells to reach their potential creating the ideal environment for positive physical change. However, taking other supplements before creating a nutritional foundation is like adding expensive accessories to a car that doesn't run properly.

Sensible supplementation is recommended in order to supply the body with the right combination of calorie-free nutrients and compounds that have the potential to enhance performance, reduce body fat, increase muscle and improve health. Proper supplementation creates the environment your body needs to get maximum results.

Inflammation

Chronic inflammation might lead to a host of diseases. There are many foods that are anti-inflammatory and inflammatory. So your food choices influence the level of inflammation within your body. As you are in the process of evaluating healthy food choices, you need to be aware of the anti-inflammatory foods and the inflammatory foods.

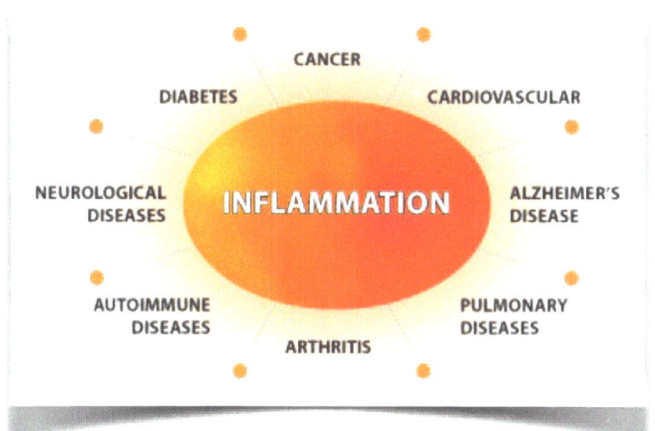

AVOID Inflammatory Foods

Sugar

Common Cooking Oils

Trans Fats

Dairy Products

Feedlot-Raised Meat

Red Meat & Processed Meat

Alcohol

Refined Grains

Artificial Food Additives

Your Personal Food Intolerances

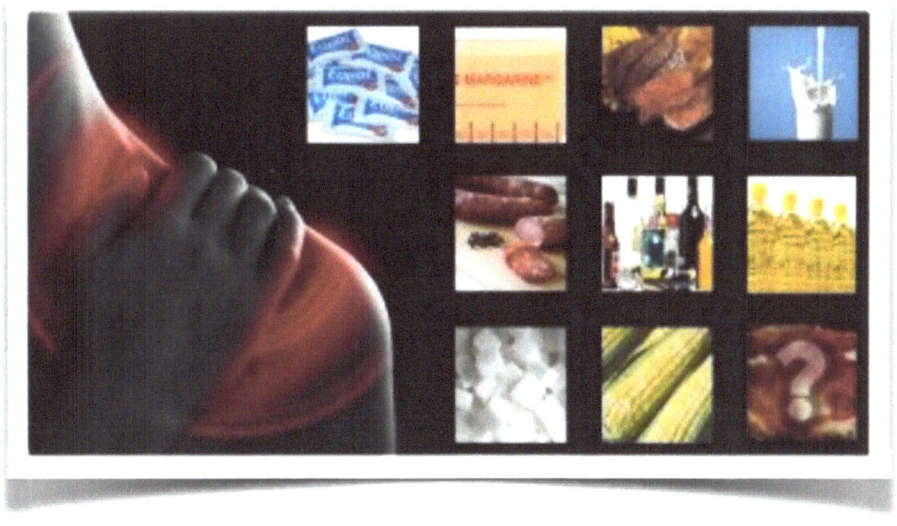

ENJOY!
Anti-Inflammatory food is what should be in your grocery cart!

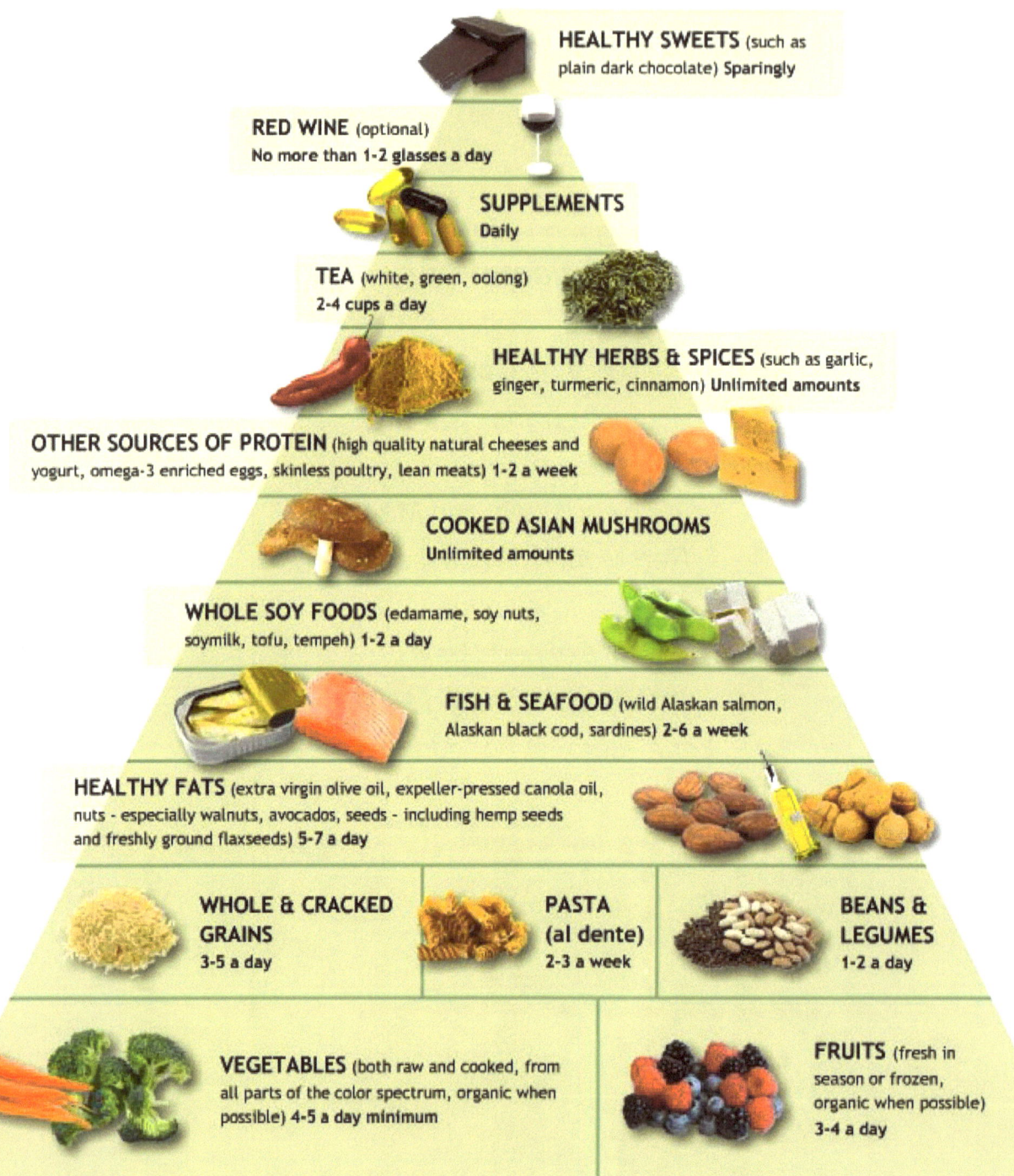

HEALTHY SWEETS (such as plain dark chocolate) Sparingly

RED WINE (optional) No more than 1-2 glasses a day

SUPPLEMENTS Daily

TEA (white, green, oolong) 2-4 cups a day

HEALTHY HERBS & SPICES (such as garlic, ginger, turmeric, cinnamon) Unlimited amounts

OTHER SOURCES OF PROTEIN (high quality natural cheeses and yogurt, omega-3 enriched eggs, skinless poultry, lean meats) 1-2 a week

COOKED ASIAN MUSHROOMS Unlimited amounts

WHOLE SOY FOODS (edamame, soy nuts, soymilk, tofu, tempeh) 1-2 a day

FISH & SEAFOOD (wild Alaskan salmon, Alaskan black cod, sardines) 2-6 a week

HEALTHY FATS (extra virgin olive oil, expeller-pressed canola oil, nuts - especially walnuts, avocados, seeds - including hemp seeds and freshly ground flaxseeds) 5-7 a day

WHOLE & CRACKED GRAINS 3-5 a day

PASTA (al dente) 2-3 a week

BEANS & LEGUMES 1-2 a day

VEGETABLES (both raw and cooked, from all parts of the color spectrum, organic when possible) 4-5 a day minimum

FRUITS (fresh in season or frozen, organic when possible) 3-4 a day

Source: Dr. Andrew Weil, MD, www.DrWeil.com

Create Your Personalized Nutritional Plan

- Establish your nutritional goals and complete the chart. *My Fitness Pal* is a great app to assist in tracking goals by calories and food categories.

Targeted Nutritional Goals	
Body weight change in pounds:	
Enter your targeted calorie count:	
Enter your change in daily calorie consumption:	
Enter your carbohydrate percent goal:	
Enter your lean protein goal:	
Enter your water consumption goal:	

Nutrition Plan

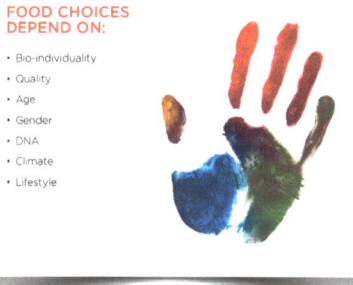

1. ***Establish your weekly menu.*** Balance your menu selections with your objectives. Select a preparation day each week to plan menus and batch-cook for your busy lifestyle.
    - Select meals that align with your goals
    - Meal planning programs are available on-line along with recipes
2. ***Shop based upon your weekly menu.***
    - Purchase only what is on your list
    - Read the label and understand the nutritional value
    - Purchase healthy clean food
    - Stock with a variety of fresh quality ingredients
    - Avoid tempting non-healthy foods
    - Do not shop when you are hungry
    - Healthier the choices, healthier the eating
3. ***Prepare your meals.***
    - Ensure that you eat based upon appropriate portions
4. ***Update your Nutrition Log***
    - Track your nutrition intake to allow you to monitor your progress and to understand where you may need to adjust your consumption

NUTRITION LOG

Day of Week: M T W Th F Sa Su	
Date _____	

Daily Goal	Calories	Protein (gr)	Carbs (gr)	Fat (gr)	Water (oz)	Comments

Actual Consumption

	Foods	Calories	Protein (gr)	Carbs (gr)	Fat (gr)	Water (oz)	Comments
Meal 1 AM PM							
Snack							
Meal 1 AM PM							
Snack							
Meal 1 AM PM							
Snack							
Total							

Juicing or Supplements

The Third Step: Exercise!

Get Active by establishing a regular workout routine. *A goal of three to five times a week for minimum of twenty minutes a day is a great start.* Progression should be your barometer; gradually increase your current fitness level. Do not fall into the trap of so many people with pushing too hard too soon. Many people get injured or become too sore and then stop within two months. Change it up so that your time exercising is interesting and you do not get bored. A balance between resistance and cardio training is important! *Overall improvements in fitness come from a combination of exercise and sound nutritional habits and a good night sleep.*

Right Choices
In making the right choices, you will notice obvious physical changes. You will notice the psychological and physiological changes as well. Expect the following:
- decreased body fat percentage
- increased lean muscle mass
- increased metabolism
- increased sense of well-being
- an abundance of energy
- lower bad and increased good cholesterol levels
- decreased risk of heart disease
- increased self-confidence and self-esteem

There is one way to achieve permanent results; follow a complete and integrated fitness program that focuses on a change in **body composition,** body fat vs. lean muscle, rather than weight. It is lean muscle that plays the key role in any type of fitness program. Whether you're interested in fat loss or muscle gain, lean muscle requires certain conditions in order to allow a positive change in body composition.

Energy In-Energy Out
To decrease fat and increase the lean muscle composition of your body you must burn more calories than the calories you take in each day. This is called creating a caloric deficit. It is the *only* way to lose fat. If you do the opposite, in other words, take in more calories than you burn, then you will gain weight. It's that simple.

Too much of anything gets stored as fat - even if you're eating nothing but healthy, nutritious foods. If you eat portions that are too large, your body will still store the extra calories as fat. Even though this appears to be a simple concept, don't be fooled. The caloric deficit must be kept small to maintain lean muscle and only lose fat weight. This strategy allows you to keep a high metabolism while at the same time transforming the shape of your body.

Weekly Meal Planner

Monday	Date
Breakfast:	
Snack:	
Lunch:	
Snack:	
Dinner:	
Side:	
Side:	
Dessert:	

Tuesday	Date
Breakfast:	
Snack:	
Lunch:	
Snack:	
Dinner:	
Side:	
Side:	
Dessert:	

Wednesday	Date
Breakfast:	
Snack:	
Lunch:	
Snack:	
Dinner:	
Side:	
Side:	
Dessert:	

Thursday	Date
Breakfast:	
Snack:	
Lunch:	
Snack:	
Dinner:	
Side:	
Side:	
Dessert:	

Friday	Date
Breakfast:	
Snack:	
Lunch:	
Snack:	
Dinner:	
Side:	
Side:	
Dessert:	

Saturday	Date
Breakfast:	
Snack:	
Lunch:	
Snack:	
Dinner:	
Side:	
Side:	
Dessert:	

Sunday	
Breakfast:	
Snack:	
Lunch:	
Snack:	
Dinner:	
Side:	
Side:	
Dessert:	

Notes

Grocery List

☐	☐
☐	☐
☐	☐
☐	☐
☐	☐
☐	☐
☐	☐
☐	☐
☐	☐
☐	☐
☐	☐
☐	☐
☐	☐
☐	☐
☐	☐
☐	☐
☐	☐

Resistance Training

Resistance training is the best way to reshape your body and get rid of unwanted fat. Want to stoke your metabolism? Start by understanding that the main tissue that burns calories is muscle, even at rest. Muscle is your furnace. The surest way to raise your metabolism and burn fat is to build and maintain muscle. The quickest way to build muscle is through resistance training.

Resistance training is performed by using weights, machines and even your own body weight to effectively work your muscles. The goal of resistance training is to gradually and progressively overload your muscles so they grow stronger. This signals your body that it's growing and healthy, not deprived and starving.

Want to burn more calories even when you are asleep? As you increase your lean body mass, you increase your metabolic rate and this makes it easier to lose fat. With a faster metabolism, you'll burn more fat all day long - even while you're sleeping!

There are numerous reasons for increasing muscle beyond making clothes fit better. One of the major benefits is in the possible prevention and rehabilitation of bone injuries. Since proper resistance training strengthens the muscles as well as the supporting structures around the joint, this form of exercise will protect our joints from the stresses of an active lifestyle.

Resistance training has many other benefits as well. You will find yourself more able to perform daily activities and move more efficiently with daily activities such as: lifting your children, carrying groceries, playing sports, moving furniture, or taking out the trash.

Form, or the correct performance of an exercise, is an important aspect of resistance training. Resistance training, if done incorrectly, can result in injury or training without results.

A program of full body resistance training, designed specifically for your body type, abilities and fitness goals for 20-45 minutes, at a minimum of 3 days per week will help you meet and exceed your goals. Allow at least one day of rest between workouts for muscle recovery and growth. Additional benefits of resistance training:
- Increased Bone Density
- Increased Lean Muscle Mass
- Increased Metabolism
- Increase Self-Esteem
- Improved Posture
- Reduces Depression
- Increased Strength

Cardio

Cardio-respiratory exercise is a term that best describes the health and function of the heart, lungs and circulatory system. This system is considered the body's transportation network for it functions by circulating blood throughout the body. The goal of any cardio workout should be to get as many large muscles working as possible. They not only need to work hard, but continuously, in order to burn the greatest amount of calories during and after exercise.

Your body quickly adapts to cardio-based workouts. The more you do, the more efficient your body becomes, causing you to burn fewer calories from your fat stores each time you exercise. Because your body adapts so quickly, cardio-lovers are forced to adjust their workouts to last increasingly longer in order to provide the same calorie burn. This not only increases the amount of time you have to spend in the gym but also increases the odds that your body may start breaking down muscle instead of fat for fuel.

FITT Principles

The most effective smart cardio programs are design around the **FITT Principles**: Frequency, Intensity, Time and Type.

Frequency

Frequency refers to the number of times cardio is performed per week. No less than three days per week, with no more than two days rest between workouts is recommended. For the first six weeks, beginners should work out every other day to prevent injury.

Intensity

Intensity is described as the speed and/or the workload of a workout. When beginning a new exercise program, a Fitness Professional can determine the intensity level most appropriate and effective for you. If you want to meet your fitness goals in the least amount of time, it is important that you continually monitor the intensity level.

Time

Time is the length of time an exercise is performed, not including warm-up and cool-down. In order to gain cardio-respiratory benefits, you may need to exercise for 20 to 30 minutes per session. It is important to remember that as you become more fit, both intensity and time can increase. Your Fitness Professional will recommend when these adjustments should be made. Remember, more is not necessarily better.

Type

Type refers to the activity used to create a stimulus. Before choosing an exercise, consider your goals, physical capacity, interests, available equipment and time constraints. Most importantly, your activity must be something that you like to do or you know will have a positive impact on your goals. Any activity that continuously uses larger muscle groups and is repetitive is best.

Create Your Personalized Exercise Plan

- Establish your exercise goals and complete the chart.

Targeted Exercise Goals	
Enter targeted calories burned:	
Enter number of cardio workouts per week:	
Enter number of cardio minutes per workout:	
Enter number of resistance workouts per week:	
Enter number of exercises and reps per workout:	

Create a weekly exercise plan that fits into your life commitments. Honor the schedule, make your exercise time an appointment on your calendar. Plan your weekly exercise plan. Planning is essential for change to happen. Planning will support your goals.

Week 1						
Monday	Tuesday	Wednesday	Thursday	Friday	Saturday	Sunday
Cardio	Upper Body Weight Training	Cardio	Lower Body Weight Training	Cardio	Upper Body Weight Training	Rest

Week 2						
Monday	Tuesday	Wednesday	Thursday	Friday	Saturday	Sunday
Cardio	Lower Body Weight Training	Cardio	Upper Body Weight Training	Cardio	Lower Body Weight Training	Rest

WORKOUT LOG

Day of Week: M T W Th F Sa Su	
Date _____	

Cardiovascular Workout

Time Spent: _____

Exercise	Time	Distances	Average HR or Intensity Level	Calories Burned	Comments

Resistance Training Workout
(Upper Lower Core)

Time Spent: _____

Exercise		1 set	2 set	3 set	4 set	5 set	6 set	Comments
	Wt							
	Rep							
	Wt							
	Rep							
	Wt							
	Rep							
	Wt							
	Rep							
	Wt							
	Rep							
	Wt							
	Rep							

Stretching

Time Spent: _____

Exercise	Duration	Comments

The Fourth Step: Sleep

Want a socially sanctioned, altered state? How about sleep? Sleep is critical to a healthy lifestyle and it is the conduit of dreams. It is the catalyst for the incredible. It is utter freedom! Through your dreams, it allows you to see what the intellect cannot. Of all the things we do on a regular basis, sleeping is one of the most extraordinary and least appreciated.

A good night's sleep rejuvenates the body and provides the energy for you to perform at your optimal level. Sleep is one of the most understated aspects of wellness and research is empirically demonstrating how critical sound and regular sleep is to physical health, mental alertness and staying even-tempered.

Sleep is a liberating state in many ways. It supports emotional freedom by refreshing your body. It's necessary for sanity and survival. It's a mini-vacation! It is as precious as oxygen, food and water. You need a break from being awake and this is what sleep provides you.

The benefits of sleep include:
- A recharged part of your brain that controls emotions.
- A sharper memory and ability to learn.
- A strengthened immune system and elevated mood.
- Beauty! That's right, when you sleep your skin cells regenerate and damage is repaired from stress, aging and ultraviolet radiation. With too little sleep, your skin doesn't renew and it looks dull. When you look marvelous, you feel marvelous!

Our sleep patterns are intimately related to the natural world. The planet turns on its axis once every twenty-four hours, giving us cycles of light and darkness, and living organisms seem to cycle with it, as seen in diurnal changes known as circadian rhythms. These rhythms show it in daily fluctuations in the release of neurotransmitters in the brain and nervous system, and in the biochemistry of our cells. We all have these basic planetary rhythms built into our systems. In fact, biologists speak of a "biological clock," controlled by the hypothalamus, a part of our brain that regulates our sleep–wake cycle which can be disrupted by things like air-travel, working the night shift, and by other behavior patterns. We cycle with the planet and our sleep pattern reflects this connection. When it is disrupted, it takes us some time to readjust, to get back to our normal sleep pattern.

Recent research from the University of Chicago has demonstrated that not getting the correct amount of sleep over time may lead to serious conditions that could compromise your health. These conditions include an impaired immune system, obesity, diabetes and high blood pressure. Inadequate sleep also may alter cognitive functioning, which is important to being successful.

In excess of 70 million Americans suffer from insomnia. Either you can't get to sleep in the first place because your thinking mind won't shut down, or you wake up in the middle of the night and you can't return to slumber. Or worse—both. The more you try to get back to sleep, the more awake you are. As it turns out, you cannot force yourself to go to sleep.

Ironically, one of the most common and earliest symptoms of stress is trouble with sleep. What are other causes of this lovely state? To name a few:
- An obsession with daily concerns that won't let your mind relax and allow sleep. Perhaps it is preoccupied with a lot of "shoulds"
- Chemical substances
- A deeper unconscious fear of loss of control, even death

If you are having difficulty sleeping, your body may be trying to tell you something. As with all other mind-body symptoms, this message is worth listening to. Most often, it is just a signal that you are going through a stressful time in your life. You can expect your sleeping pattern to improve by itself. Sometimes it helps to look at how much exercise you are getting. Regular exercise, such as walking or yoga or swimming, can make a major difference in your ability to sleep soundly, as you can discover by experimenting for yourself.

Sometimes people get caught up in the thinking that they need more sleep than they really do. Our need for sleep changes as we grow and is known to diminish as we get older. Some people can function well on four hours of sleep per night, but they may feel that they "should" be able to sleep longer. Others need the seven or eight hours normally prescribed.

Often times, it is our great attachment to sleep that causes us to worry about the consequences of losing sleep. Hmmmmmmm. Paradigm shift, if you shift to the belief that your body and mind can self- regulate and correct for some of these disturbances we experience, then you can use your sleep imbalance as a vehicle for further growth, just as we have seen that you can use other symptoms, even pain or anxiety, to come to deeper levels of wholeness.

As stated earlier, balance is not a math equation and neither is the amount of sleep you need or what time of the day or night sleep works best for you. It all depends on you. People are different and they have different rhythms. Some function best late at night, others function best early in the morning. It's very useful to examine how you might use the twenty four hours you have each day in the way that works best for you. You can only do this by listening carefully to your mind and body and letting them teach you what you need to know. This means letting go of the idea that less sleep means less life. That may not be so for you.

If we make a commitment to ourselves to be fully awake when we are awake, then our view of not being able to sleep at certain times will change along with our view of everything else. Whenever we happen to be awake in the twenty-four hour cycle can be seen as an opportunity to practice being fully awake and accepting things as they are, including that your mind is agitated and that you are unable to sleep. When you do this, more often than not, your sleep pattern will take care of itself. However, don't be surprised when it doesn't come when you think it should or for as long as you think it should. So much for the "shoulds."

When you can't sleep, get out of bed and do something else for awhile. This can be something that you like to do or that you might feel good about getting done. Some people meditate, others read a good book, others work on projects. The key is to be fully awake.

Here are some additional tips for conquering the insanity of insomnia:
- Several hours prior to going to sleep, avoid sleep thieves like excess alcohol, sugar, a large meal or too many drinks that can lead to a full bladder.
- Avoid emotional stimulation like arguments, discussing charged emotional issues, violent newscasts, or stressful chores like paying bills.
- Breathe - when you are tense, you tend to hold your breath and grind your teeth. How unattractive is that? Deeply breathe in and breathe out. Exhale the toxicity of all of your worry, panic and fear. Lull yourself to sleep by focusing on your breath's hypnotic rhythm.
- Serenity Now! Repeat the serenity prayer. If you are kept up by a problem which it's possible you may not even remember a month from now, or escalating anxiety, say this prayer as needed to release the stress:
    > God, grant me the serenity to accept the things that I cannot change, the courage to change the things I can, and the wisdom to know the difference.

Helpful tips for getting yourself on a routine of good sleep include:
- Establish a sleep routine with the same time daily for going to bed and getting up in the morning.
- Do a relaxing, quiet activity such as reading, a warm bath or listening to soothing music shortly before going to bed.
- Set aside a brief amount of time to worry daily, and when the time is up, stop worrying and go on with your daily tasks.
- Regular daily exercise - aside from many other wonderful health benefits, usually makes it easier to fall asleep and sleep better. As little as twenty to thirty minutes of activity helps. A brisk walk, a bicycle ride or a run is time well spent. However, be sure to schedule your exercise in the morning or early afternoon. Exercising too late in the day actually stimulates the body, raising its temperature. That's the opposite of what you want near bedtime, because a cooler body temperature is associated with sleep.

Interference to Sleep
- Napping during the day can interfere with sleep.
- If you need to nap, do it in the early afternoon and sleep no longer than 30 minutes.
- Alcohol reduces overall quality of sleep.
- Caffeine can cause sleep problems up to 10 -12 hours after drinking it.
- Smoking - nicotine is a stimulant which disrupts sleep.

Preparing for Sleep
- Foods that help you sleep
  - Glass of warm milk and half a turkey or peanut butter sandwich
  - Whole-grain, low-sugar cereal or granola with low-fat milk or yogurt
  - Banana and a cup of hot chamomile tea

Develop a relaxing bedtime routine
- Consistent, relaxing routine before bed sends signal to your brain to rest
- Warm bath, soft music, quiet reading
- Yoga
- Muscle relaxation

Bedroom
- Master the art of picking a great mattress.
- Get luxurious sheets, blankets and comforters.
- Sleep in a room that is cool, dark and quiet.
- Use a white noise box or a relaxation tape to help you sleep if noises disturb you.
- Internal body clock helps regulate sleep and can be sensitive to light and dark.
- Free flow of air!

Sleep - your mind, your body and your spirit are the recipients of its grace. You'll gather input about keeping your total self in mint condition. When you go to sleep, you go to the big show. Every night is opening night.

The Fifth Step: Accountability

A program customized for you will improve your results. When you combine an effective fitness program with proper nutrition, supplements and accountability, you can make incredible changes, but it must be made of things that you love, from exercise to the foods that you are eating. To be successful the changes need to be lifestyle changes.

Research shows that specific, scheduled accountability check-ins with another person or group increases your chances of actually doing something by 85 percentage points! Get a buddy!

Your accountability pal can be anyone, a family member, a friend or a coach, and your way of checking in must work for both of you. Does an email listing of all that you have accomplished over the past week work for you? Does a quick phone call work for you?

In any case, it's worth it to have regular check-ins with someone in order to:
- Keep yourself accountable.
- Acknowledge progress and recognize what you are learning about yourself, your behavior patterns and what works well in your life.
- To celebrate your successes!
- Keep you going when times are tough!

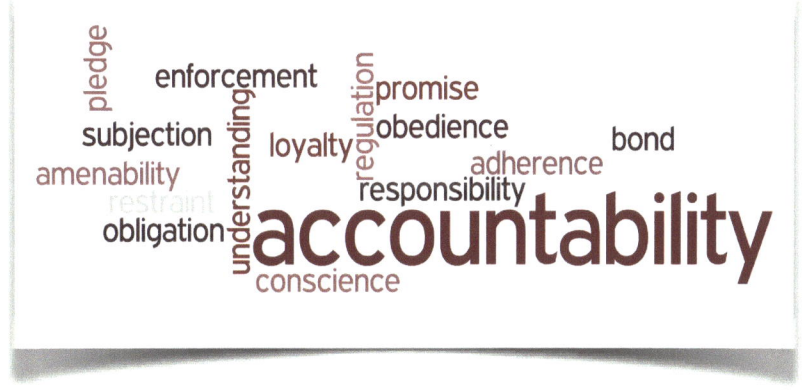

Live Life Well

To Change You Must Change. Lifestyle Change! It's time to take responsibility for creating the wellness you desire. It's time to start creating new habits. It is time to achieve your goals.

Strategy Review for Weight Change
- Set reasonable weight goals, healthy loss or gain of 1-2 pounds weekly is a good gauge.
- Focus on lowering your fat intake, balance your choices over several days.
- Get physical, let a variety of fun activities help shape your daily routine.
- Use the buddy system, a walking buddy or a low-fat cooking partner can be inspiring.
- Build on the positive, learn from your lapses and reward your changes.
- Redefine success, energy, esteem, and health are benefits that can't be measured on the scale but are extremely important.

The Power of Habit
Success and failure are simply habits, and the good news is that good habits are just as difficult to break as bad ones. Good habits are hard to establish but easy to live with and bad habits are easy to establish and hard to live with. Motivation gets us started on the road to success and good habits are the fuel that keeps us making progress. Just as bad habits can lead to a downward spiral, good habits escalate and lead to an upward spiral.

Welcome the challenges that face you. With effort and patience you have the full potential to create a positive change with your physique and your quality of life. There are only three conditions necessary for the acquisition of any new habit or skill. The COURAGE to try something you do not know how to do, the PATIENCE to try again once you have discovered that you don't know how to do it and the PERSEVERANCE to keep trying, as many times as necessary, until you do know how to do it.

To Destination-Success!
Enjoy this life-changing journey by accepting and living by the basic understanding that this material is built around the premise of progress, not perfection. Your perfect size and shape may not match that of your friend's perfect size and shape.

Give yourself credit for baby-steps. By developing awareness that improvement is measured by your daily progress, you can save yourself a lot of grief and frustration from the beginning. Focusing on small, positive steps in everything you do is a vital component to a permanent physical change. With time, commitment and a willingness to continue to take those small steps, failure is not an option.

Allow yourself a break from your new focus 10% of the time. 90% of the time keep the focus and you will accomplish your goals!

The following steps will ensure that you receive the maximum benefit from your experiences. They will play an essential role in helping you achieve your goals of ultimate leanness and energy. Improvement will become apparent in a matter of weeks.

- **Decide on what you want to achieve** – Have a clear vision of the end result. Close your eyes and visualize your ideal body. Picture exactly how you look, size and shape you are and how you feel.
- **Know and feel your REASON** for wanting to achieve these particular results – Continue to ask yourself "why" until you elicit an emotional response.
- **Believe you are capable and deserving** of reaching this goal – If others can do it, why can't you?
- **Make this a priority** in your life, every day. Schedule workouts, schedule your meals, keep kitchen stocked with healthy clean food.
- **Start taking actions** that bring results – each day strive to do something a little better than the day before.
- **Be grateful** - understand that the quickest way to achieve my goals is to be happy NOW.
- **Be forgiving** - If you slip, quickly return to your plan. Don't feel guilty, but remain enthusiastic about the process and with myself.

Empowering yourself and optimizing your energy to live a balanced, healthier and fuller life every day!

LIVE LIFE WELL!

Lori Vargas, MBA, CPA, Health Coach, is the founder of *Spa Vargas Wellness,* built upon the mission statement to provide a memorable experience with therapeutic benefits. Lori's philosophy is to enjoy the journey and the destination which is her tag line and life pursuit.

She founded *Vargas Consulting* which directs spa development, consults with spa entrepreneurs, and operates three successful locations in the Midwest.

She found *Spa Vargas University School of Massage Therapy*, educating students on becoming business-mined and nurturing massage therapists.

Lori is an Adjunct Professor at the College of Dupage where she teaches Entrepreneurship, Spa Management and Resort Management.

Prior to becoming an entrepreneur, Lori served in corporate finance in Fortune 50 firms. She holds an MBA from the University of Chicago.

As a mother of two boys, she strives to create a balanced life and always pursues living in the present. Her children are her inspiration and she is grateful to them for the happiness they bring to her life.